✿

This is dedicated to my grandma Audrey who sadly passed of breast cancer.

✿

https://themonster-series.com

Illustrations by Dmitry Chizhov

Thanks to author Karen McMillan for her assistance with this project.

ISBN: 978-1-9162194-0-3

In collaboration with Duckling Publishing and Chrissy Metge Ltd.
www.ducklingpublishing.com
www.chrissymetge.com

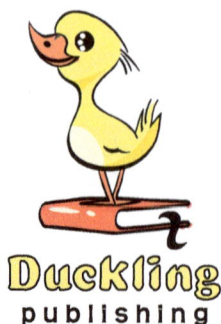

Duckling
publishing

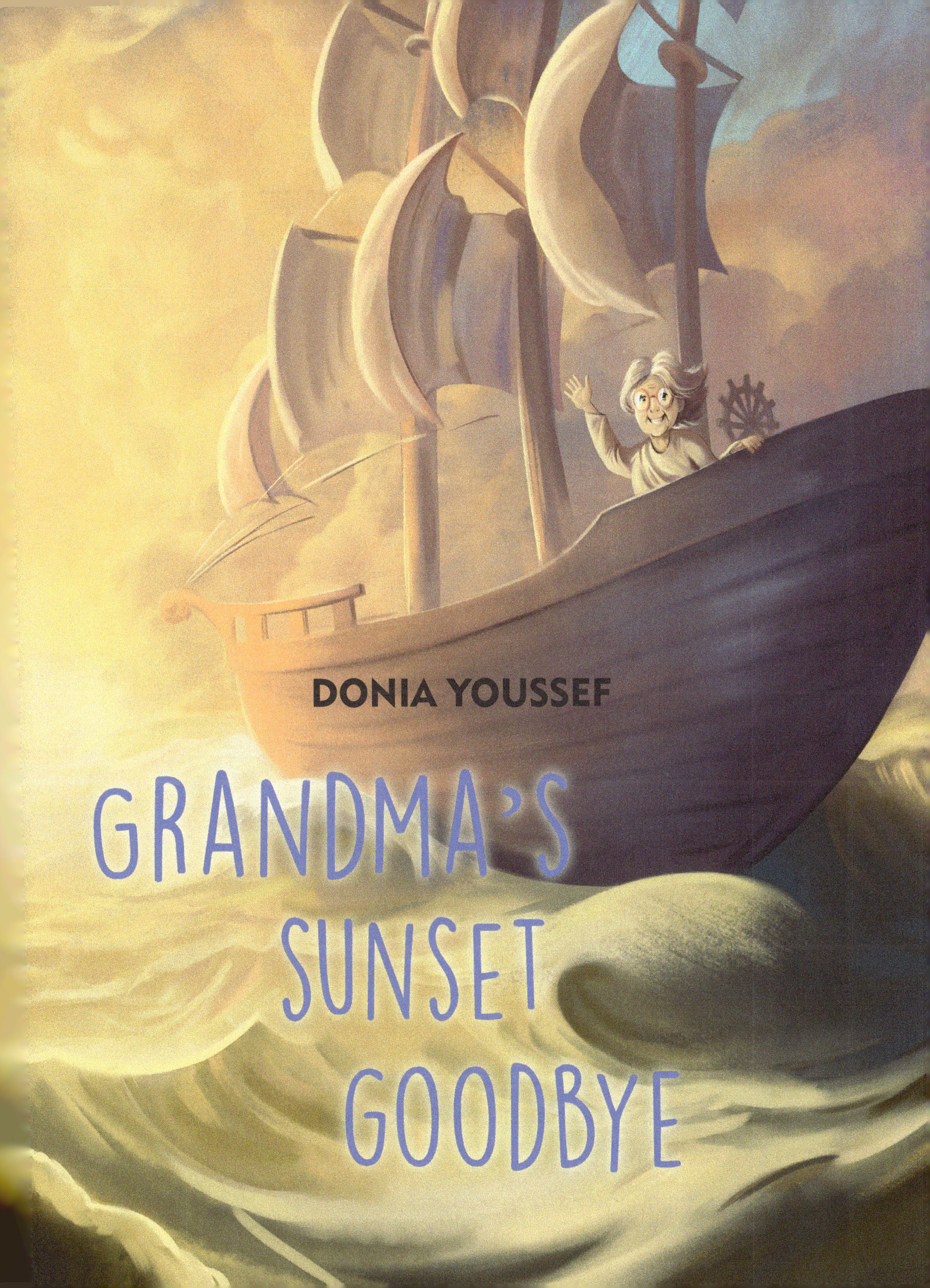

DONIA YOUSSEF

GRANDMA'S SUNSET GOODBYE

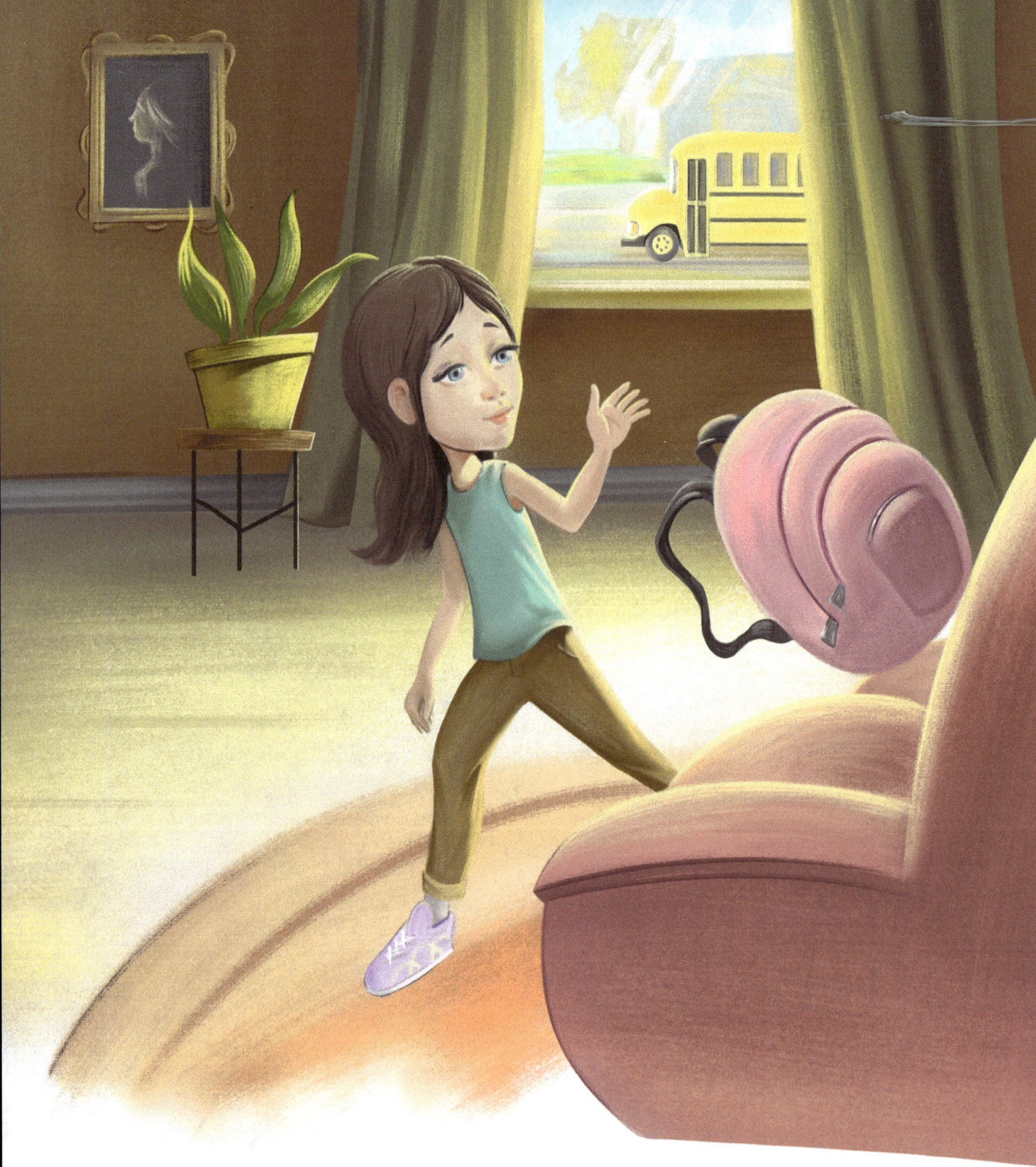

Katie came home from school and tossed her backpack on the couch. She planned to do her homework after getting an apple to eat from the kitchen.

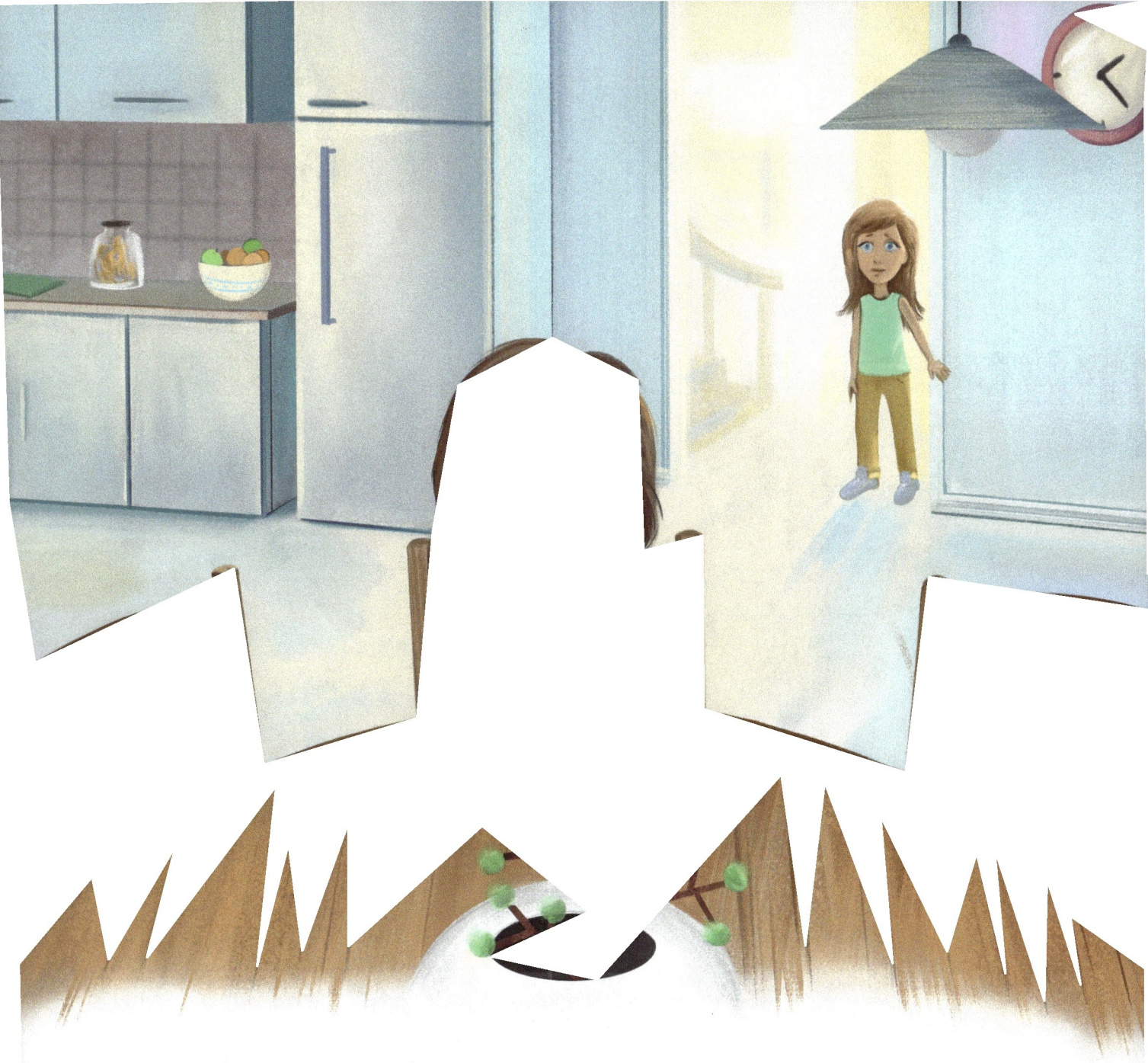

When she went to the kitchen, Katie found Mummy sitting at the table with her head in her hands.

'What's wrong, Mummy?' asked Katie.

Mummy wiped a few tears from her face.
'Give me a hug,' said Mummy. Katie hugged Mummy.
'What happened, Mummy?' she asked.

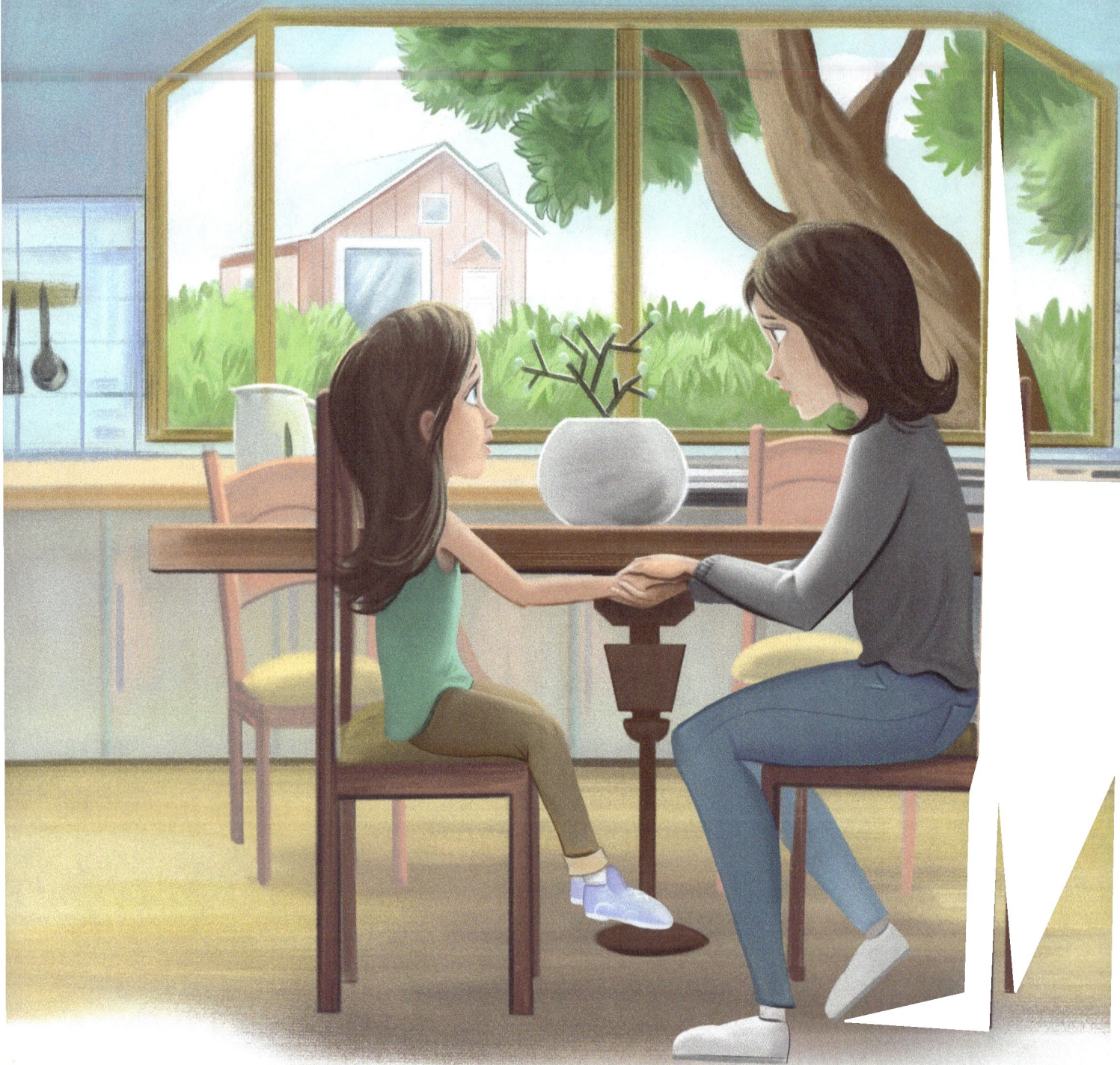

'Sit down, Katie.' Mummy patted the chair beside her.
'I have something to tell you. Grandma passed away last night.'

Katie shook her head. 'What do you mean?'

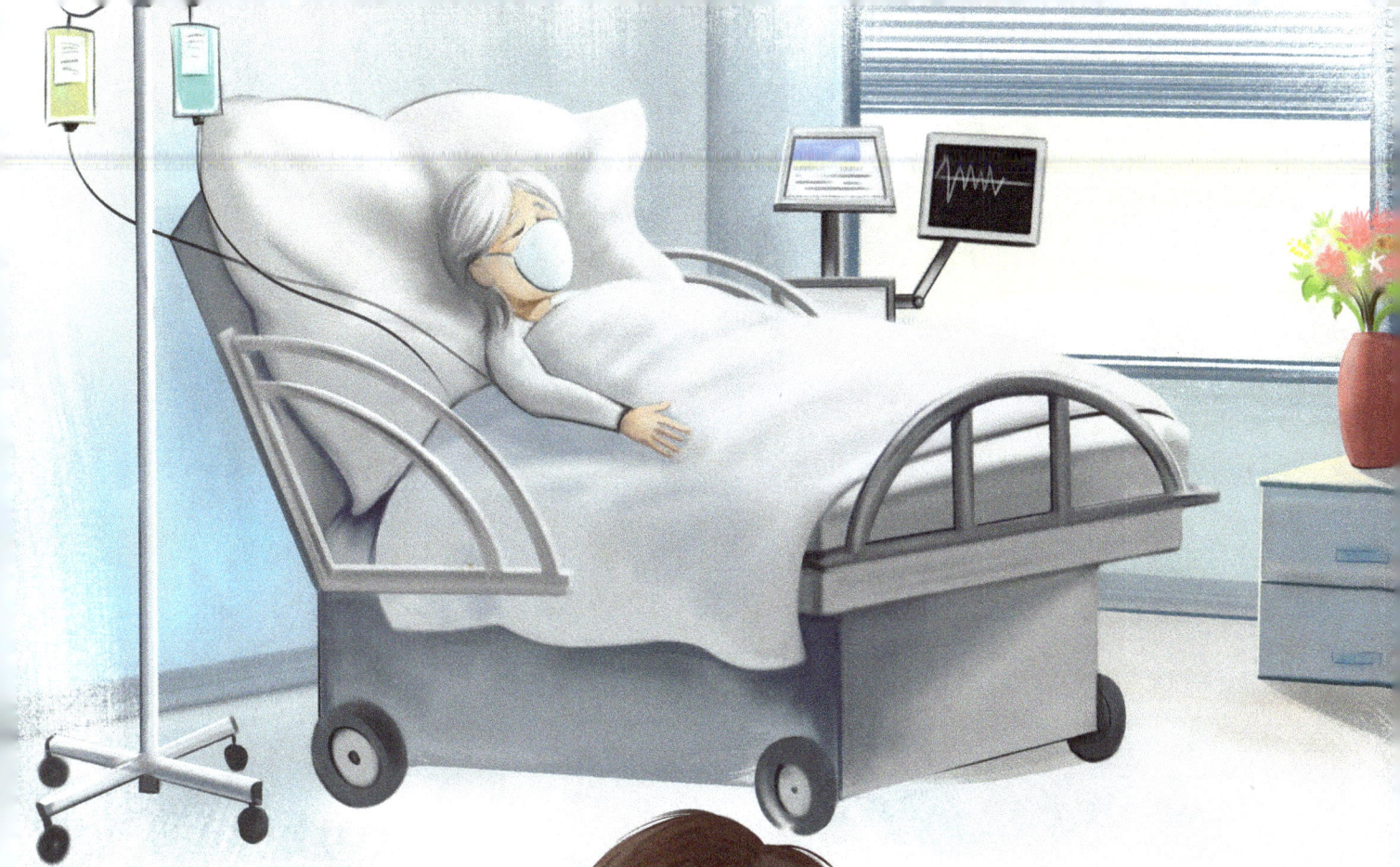

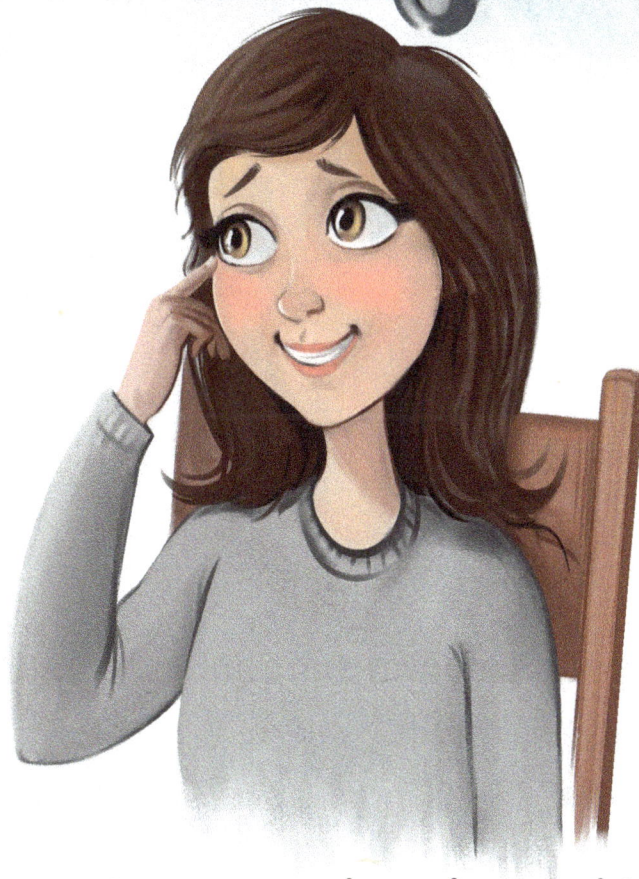

Mummy's eyes were watery even when she tried to smile.
'As you know, Grandma had cancer, and last night she slipped into a coma. She died last night.'

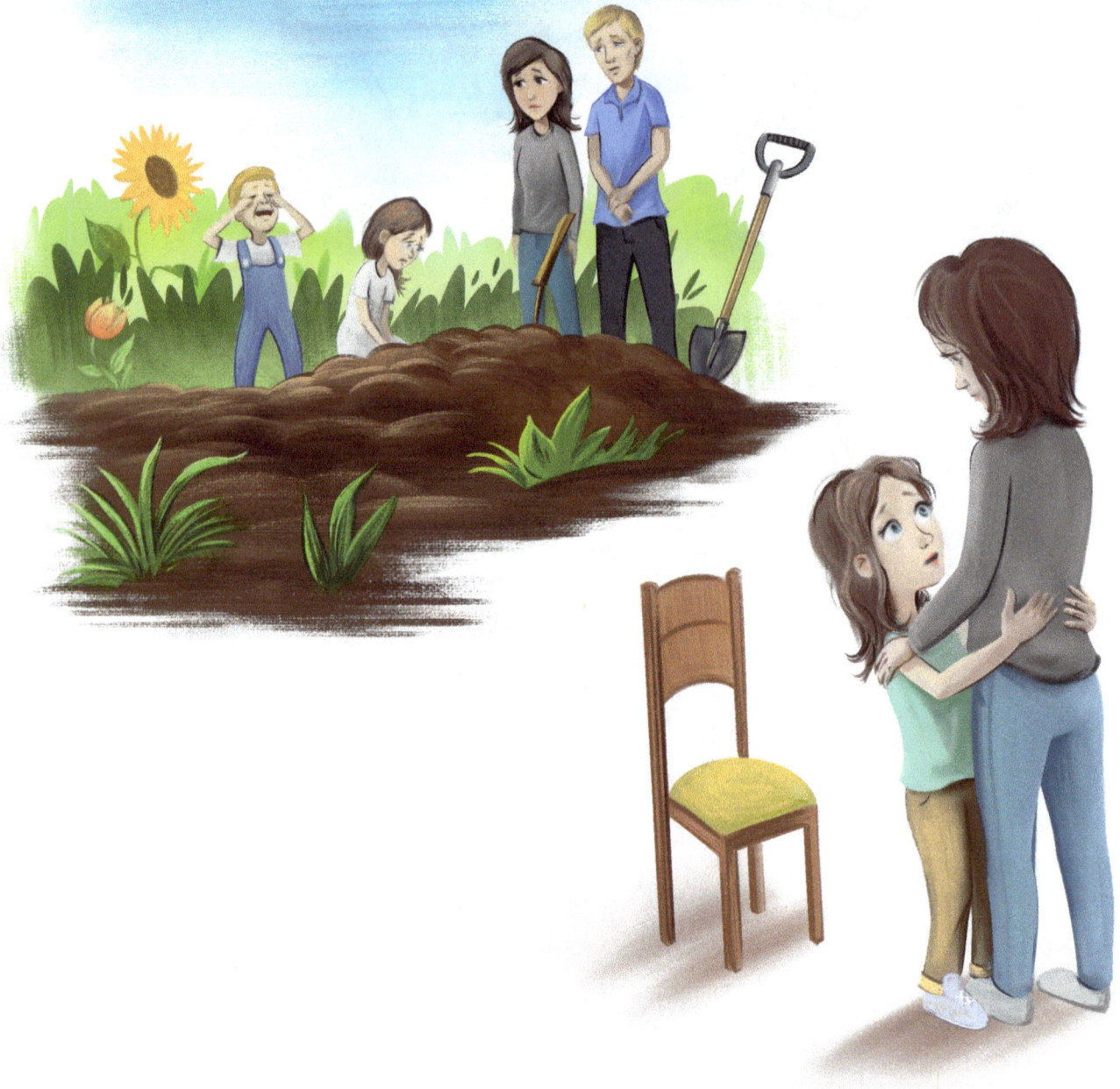

Katie felt her heart flutter, and suddenly she felt like crying too.
She and Mummy hugged again.
'But is she really gone? Like Charlie?' asked Katie.

Charlie was Katie's pet turtle who passed away last year. Katie, her
brother Richard, and Mummy and Daddy buried Charlie under the
oak tree in the backyard.

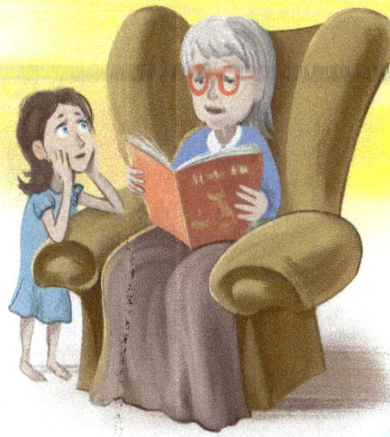

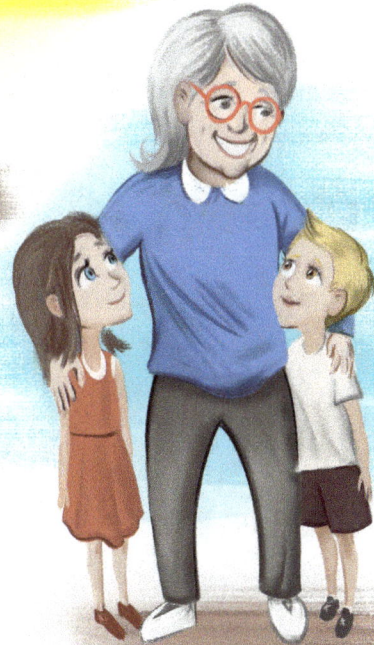

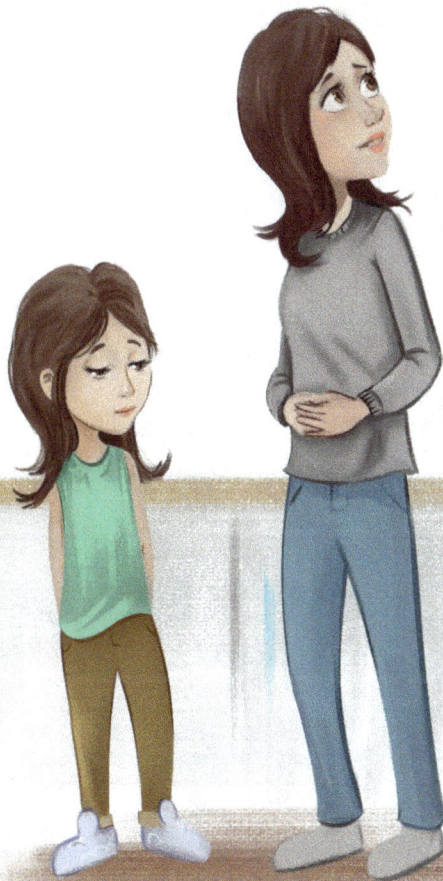

'That's right, sweetheart,' Mummy said. 'We expected something like this to happen. It's sad but remember that Grandma lived a long full life with us. It was her time to go.'

Katie nodded. 'I understand. I'm still sad, though.'

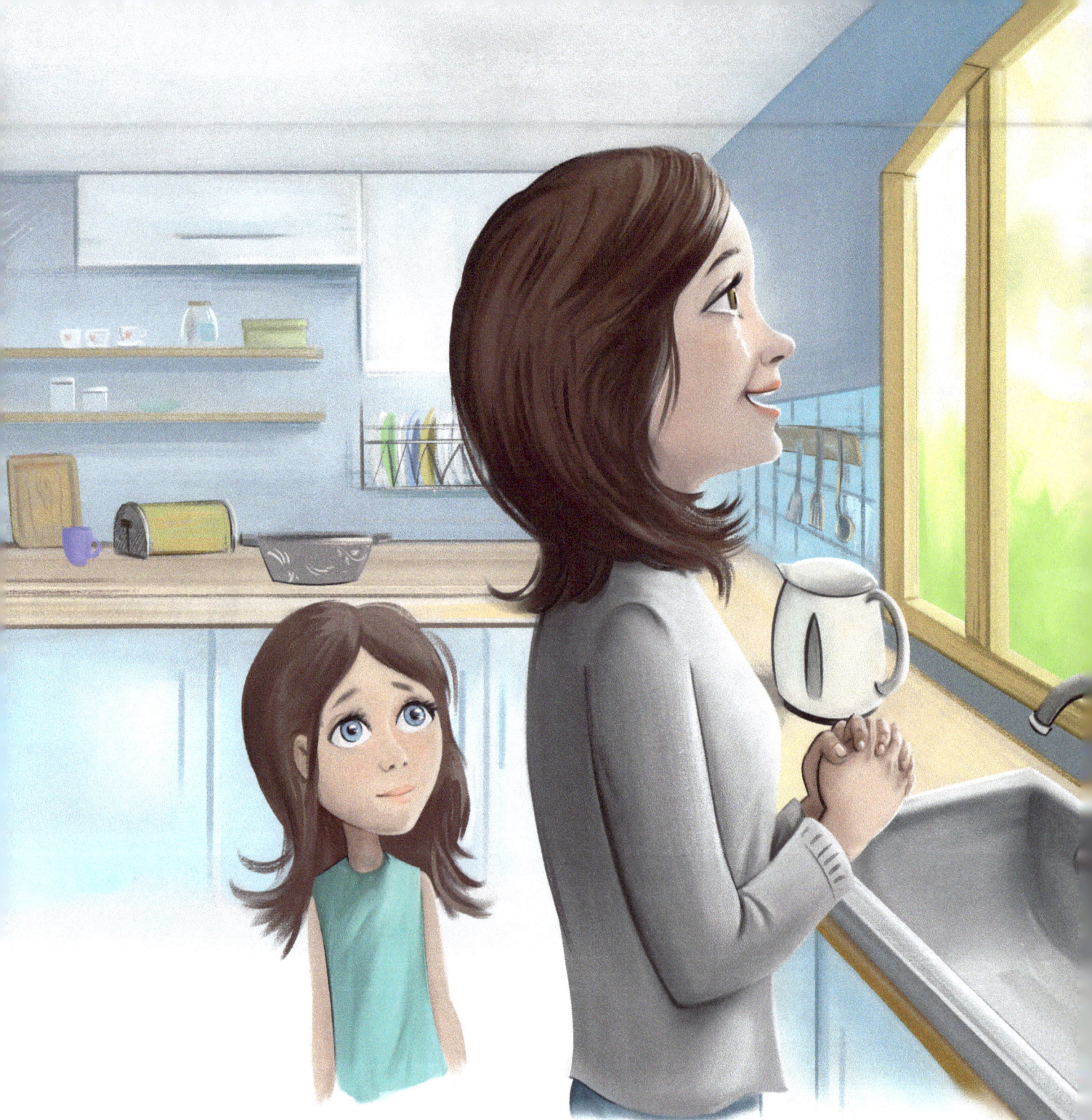

Mummy laughed, and more tears rolled down her cheeks. 'I know, I am too, Katie. It's normal to have so many feelings, especially sadness, when someone you love so much, who is so close to you, passes away like this.'

'Even when you expect it?' Katie asked.

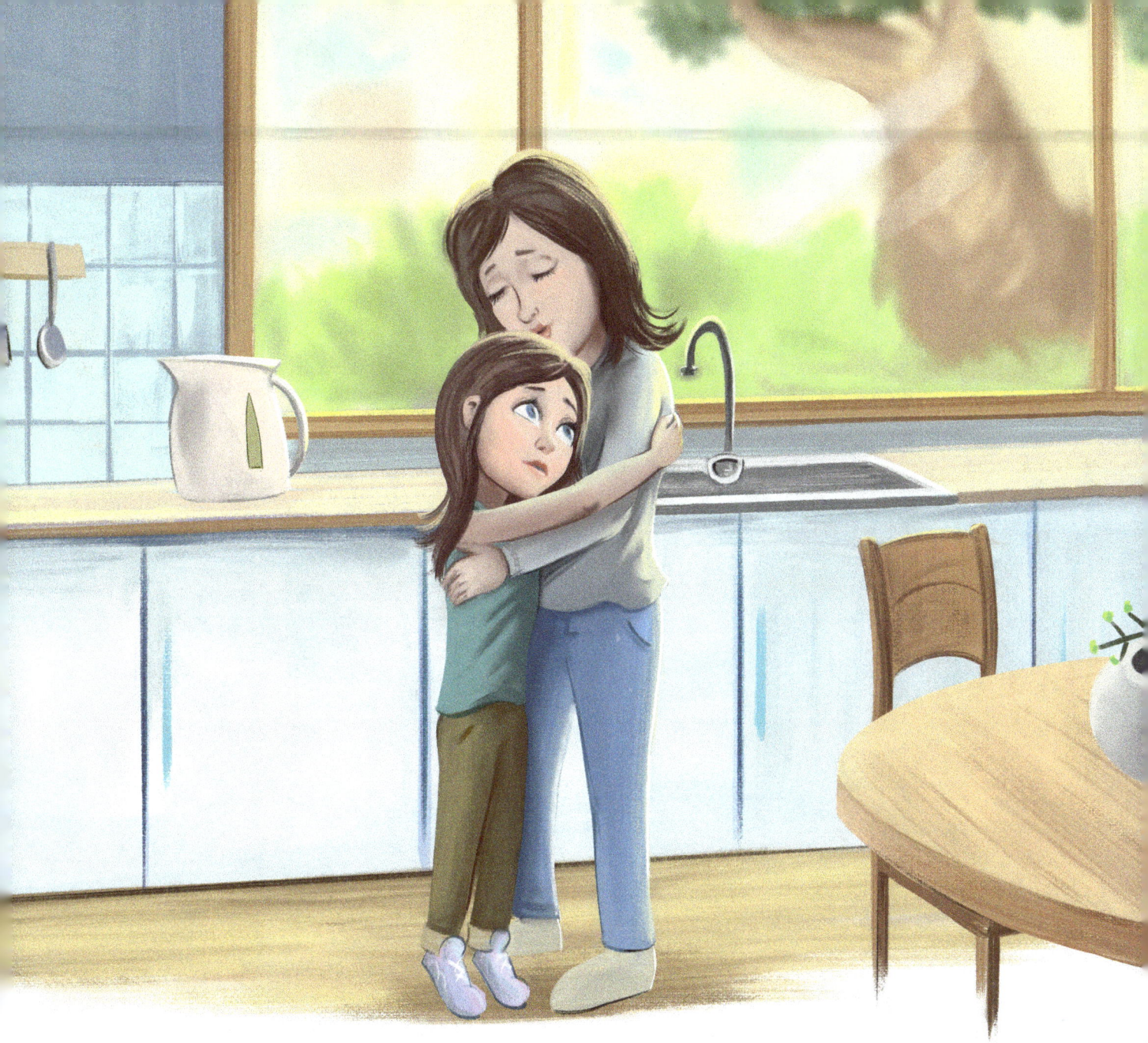

'Oh yes, even when you expect it.' Mummy wiped her tears. 'When someone passes, you miss them so much, and so many feelings run through your mind, and you feel it all over.'

'You remember them.' Katie said.

'That's right'. Mummy hugged Katie again. 'You remember all the good times with them. Even the sad ones, too. And the funny ones.'

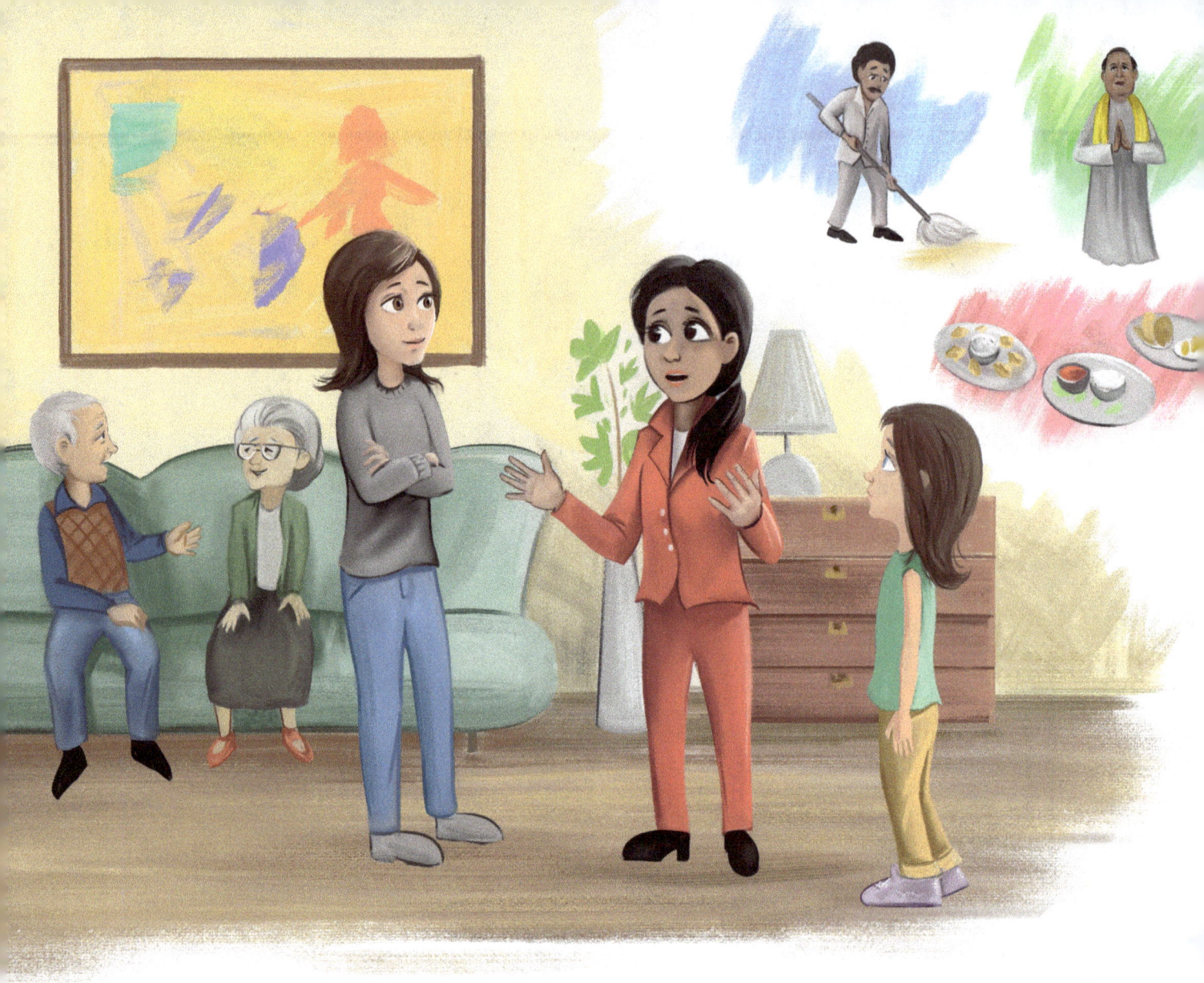

Mummy made plans for Grandma's Christian funeral, and many of Mummy's friends came to visit during this time. People wanted to know about the plans for Grandma's funeral, and people shared about how they handle death in their own culture also.

One friend said, 'I'm Hindu, and in my tradition, we clean our house after someone passes away, wash, and our priest says a special prayer afterward. We also eat sweet foods and say goodbye to our loved one and remember all the kind things they did.'

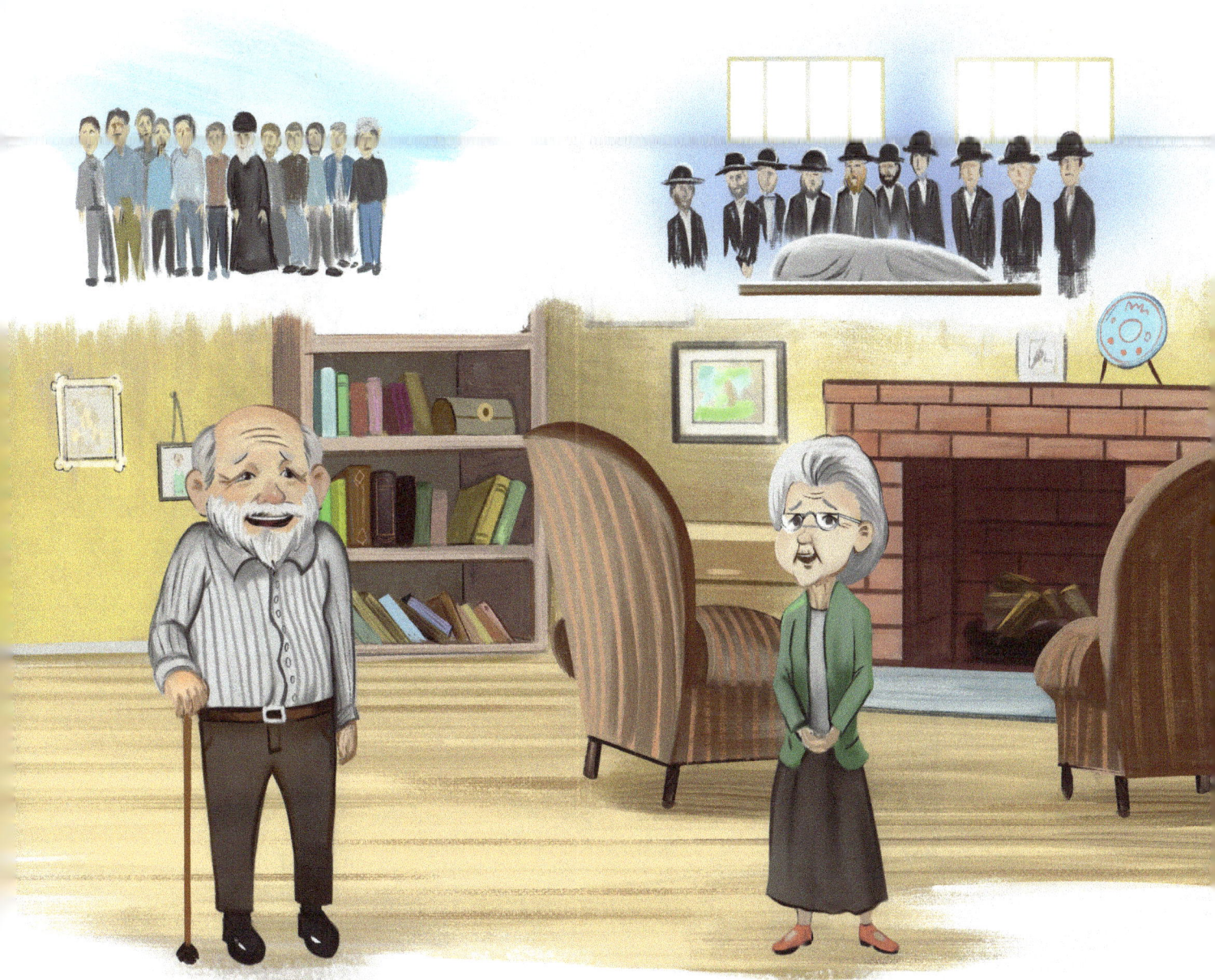

An old friend of Grandma said, 'I'm Muslim, and we say special prayers after someone passes, outside of our mosques, facing toward Mecca. It is called Salat al-Janazah'.

Another friend said, 'I'm Jewish, and the funeral is followed by a seven-day mourning period called the Shiva where all the family and their friends gather to remember their loved one.'

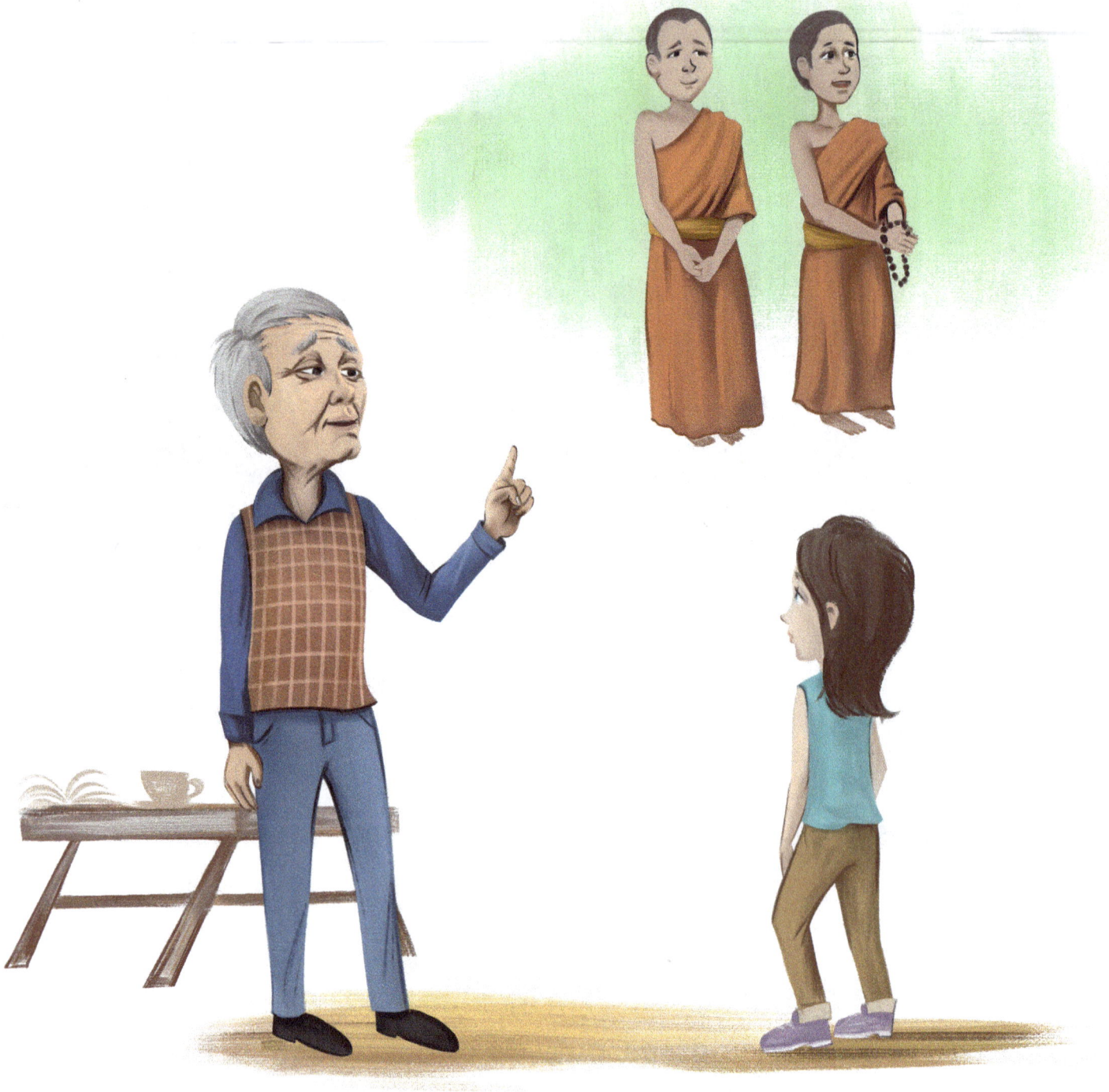

Another friend said, 'I'm Buddhist, and we offer words of goodwill to the person who has passed in our ceremony, encouraging them to let go of worldly things.'

Katie listened with interest to their stories and thought they were all wonderful things.

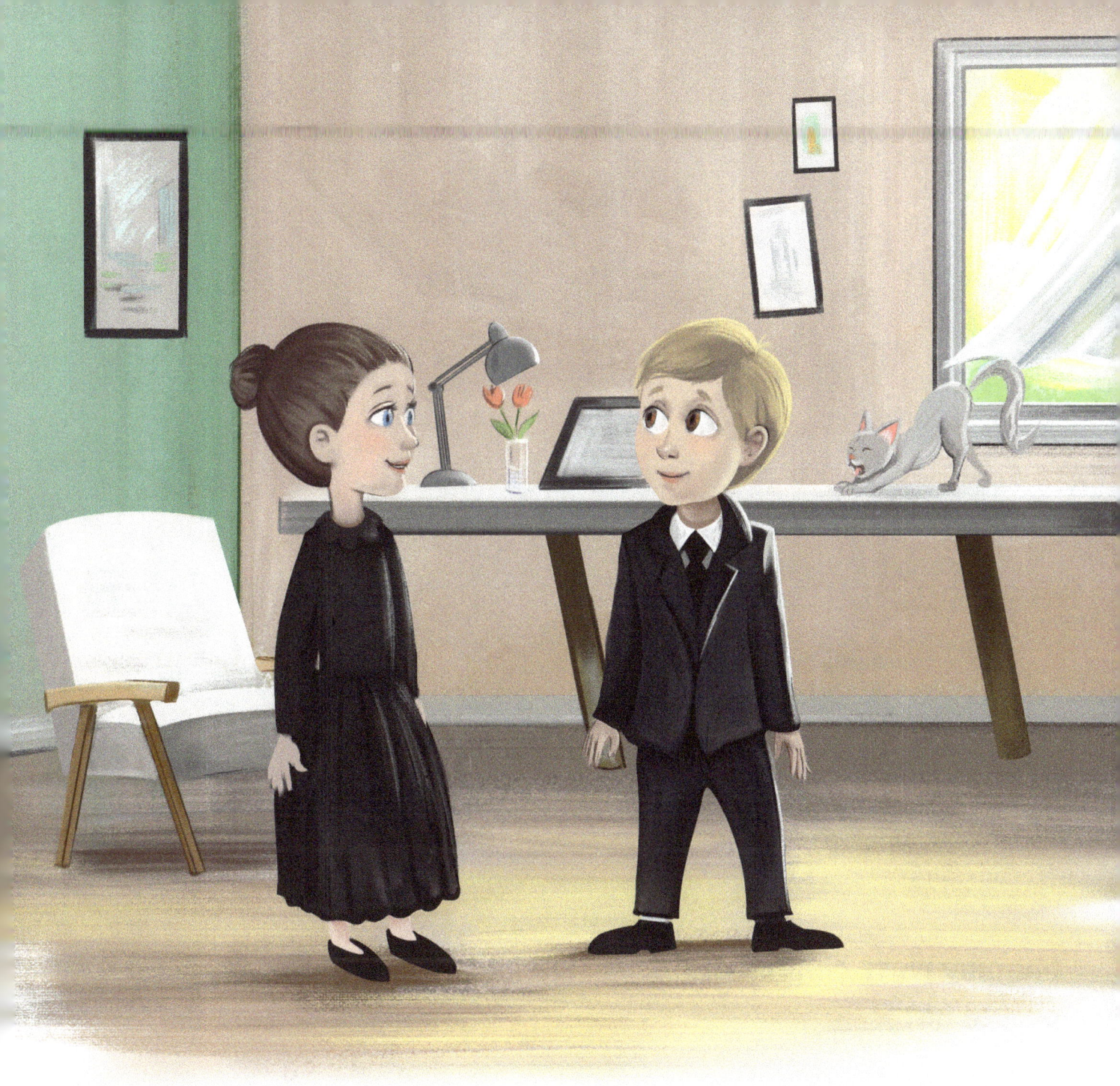

The day of the funeral arrived, and everyone in the family, all their friends, and Grandma's friends were invited.

Katie and her little brother Richard got dressed for the funeral. They wore nice clothes: Katie in a black dress and Richard in his suit.

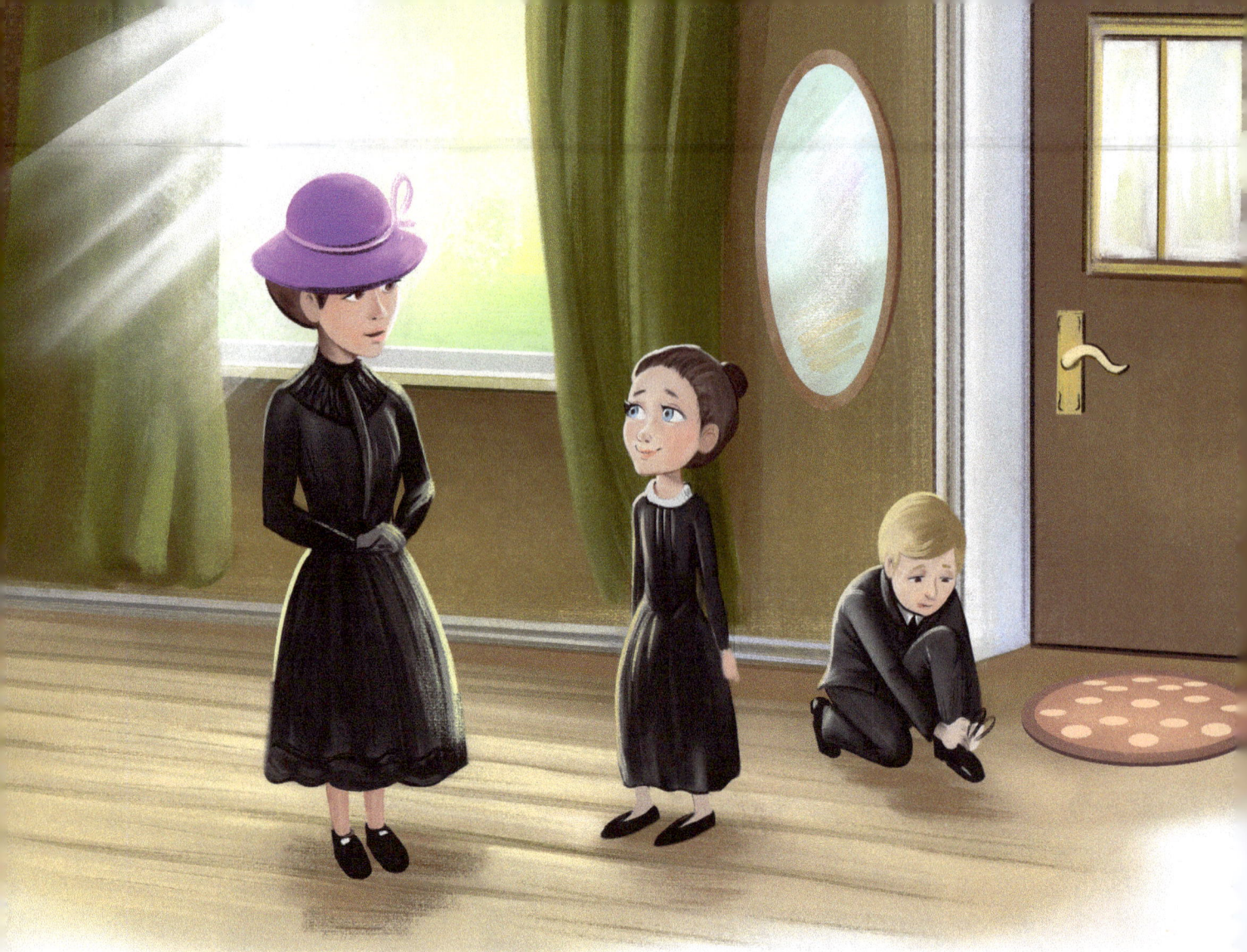

Mummy wore a black dress, but she also wore a colourful purple hat.

'Grandma, my mum, always said she didn't want people to cry at her funeral,' said Mummy.

Katie smiled. 'Grandma was so nice, but she knew people would be sad, right?'

Mummy said, 'Oh yes, but she wanted them to remember the good times with her.'

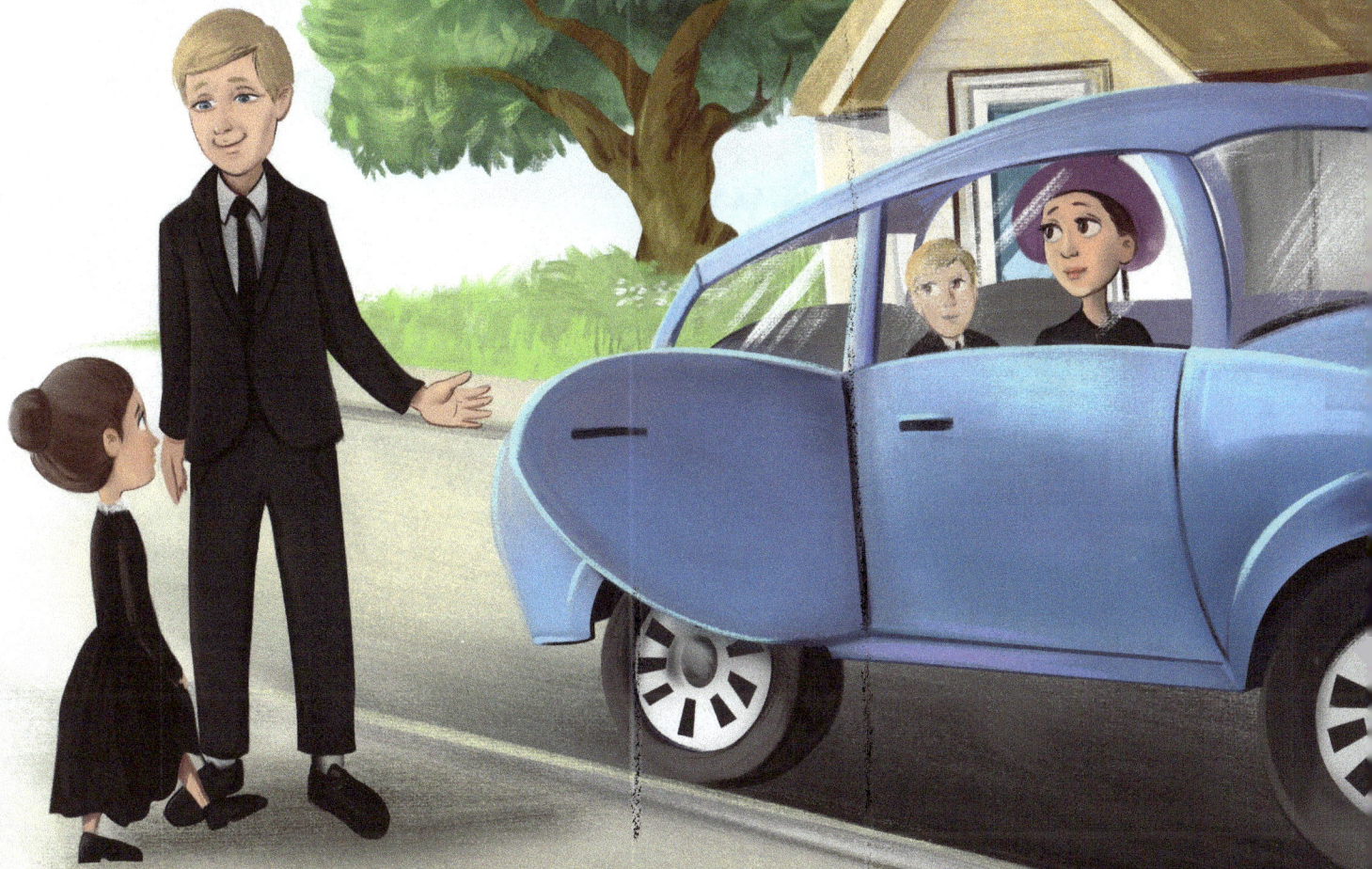

Daddy came in and he wore a black suit too. 'Are we ready?'

Everyone got into the car and drove to the funeral home.

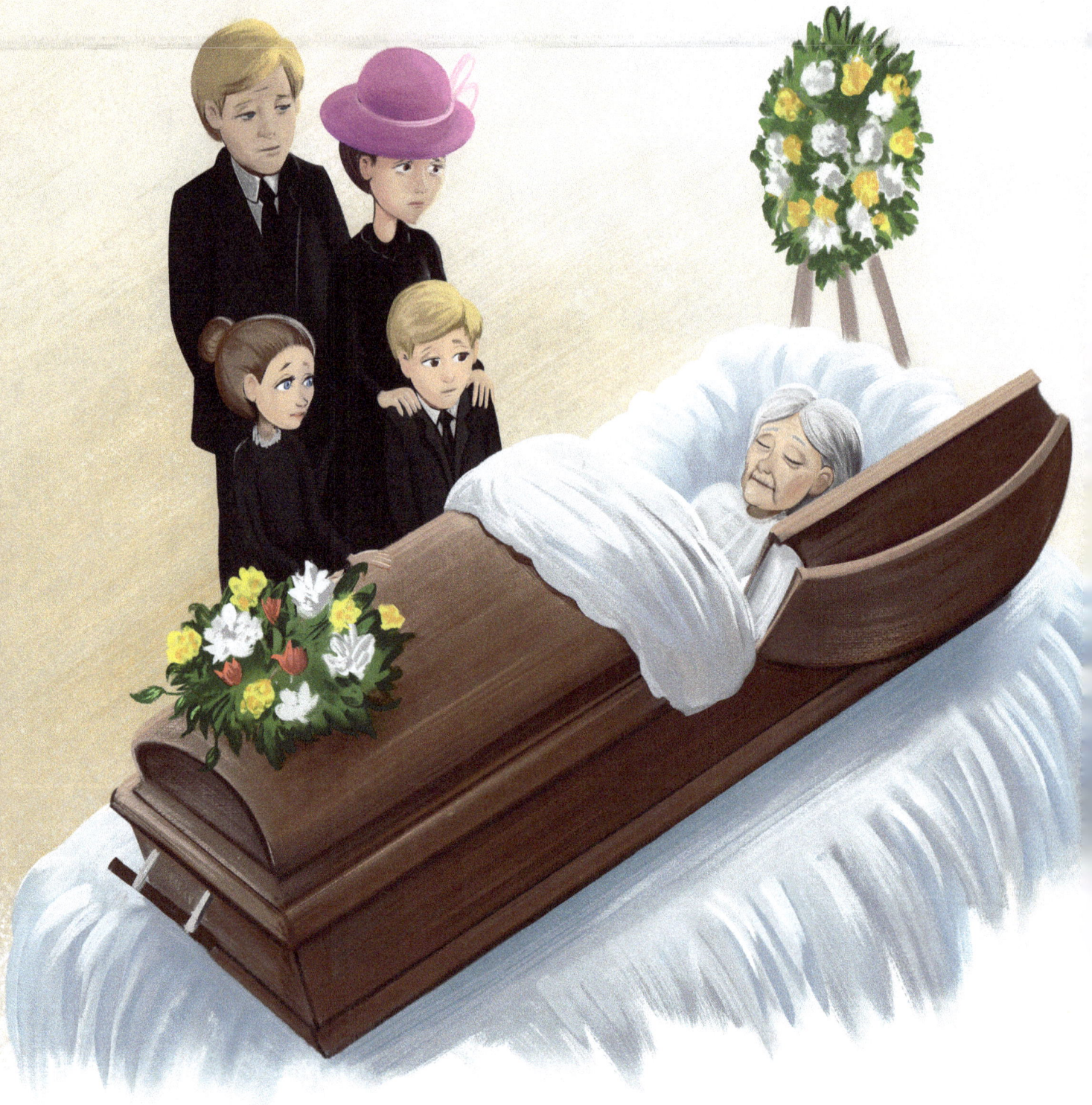

At the funeral home they saw Grandma and she looked asleep.

'She looks so peaceful,' Katie said. 'I can't believe she's gone.'

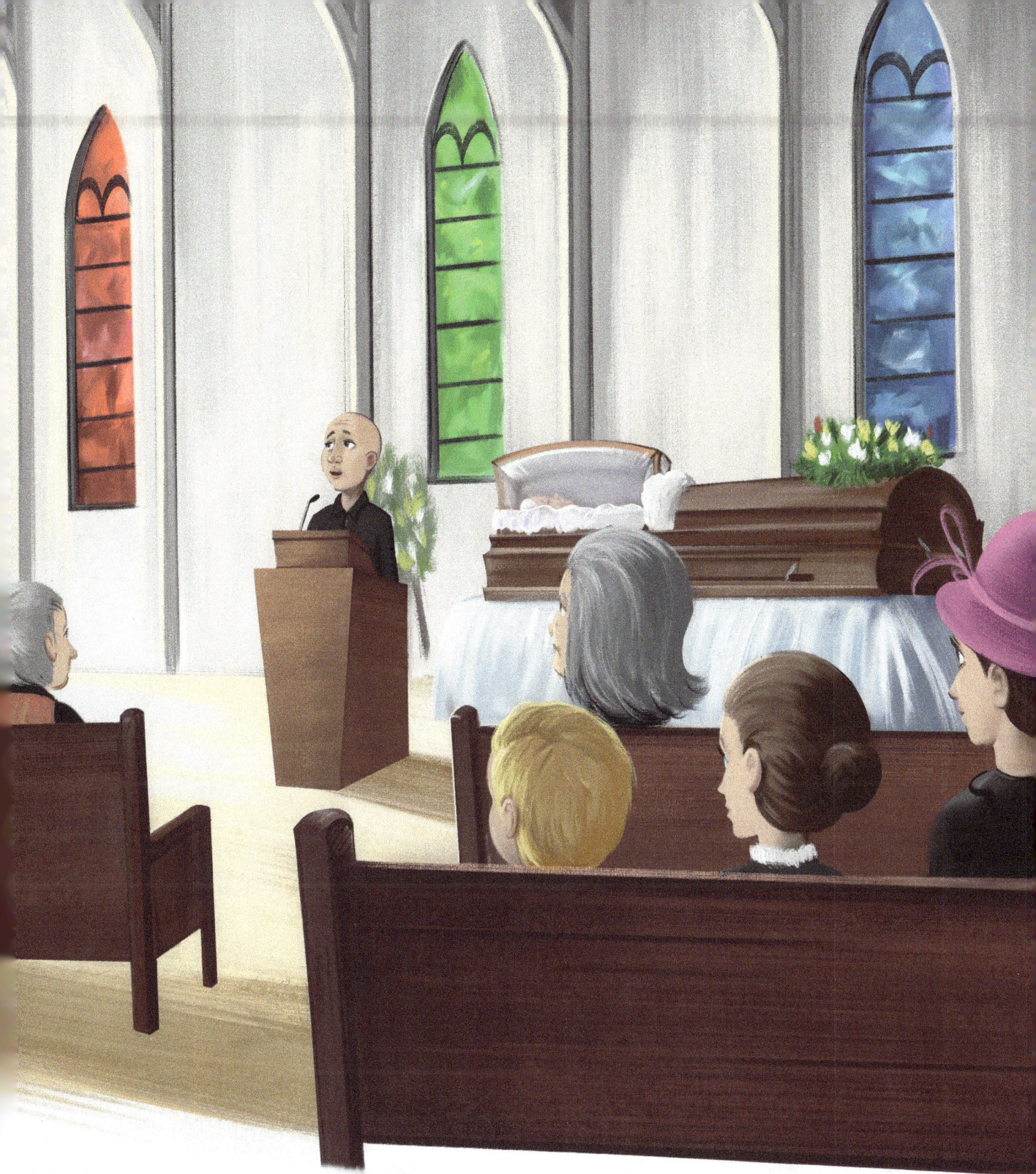

Many people spoke at Grandma's wake, which is where people can talk about whoever passed away. They told many happy and funny stories about Grandma.

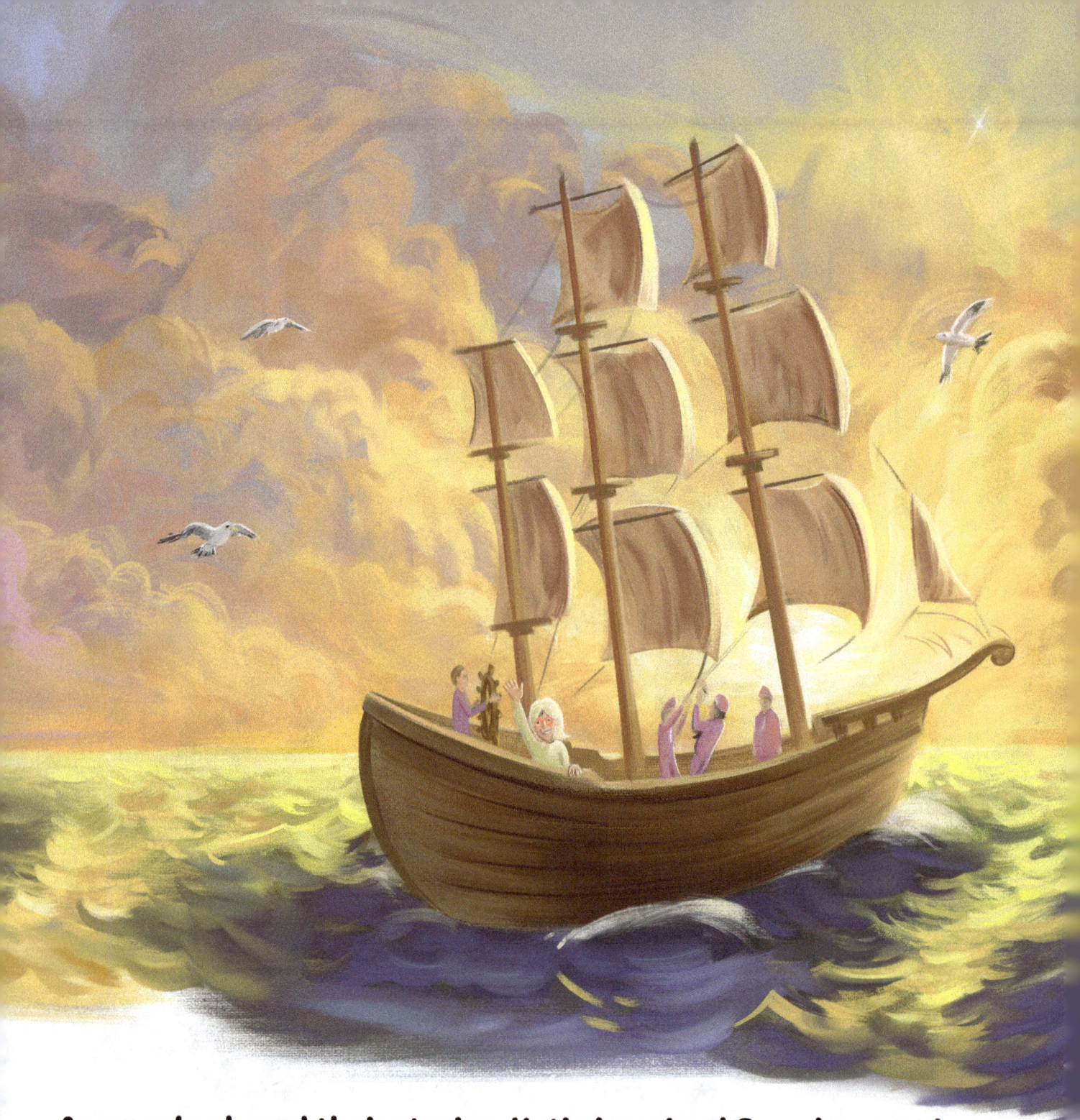

As people shared their stories, Katie imagined Grandma waving at everyone and getting onto a big boat. The boat had big white sails and a crew of people dressed in colourful uniforms. When they set sail and drifted off into the sunset, Grandma, in Katie's imagination, waved and said goodbye. And Grandma had a smile on her face.

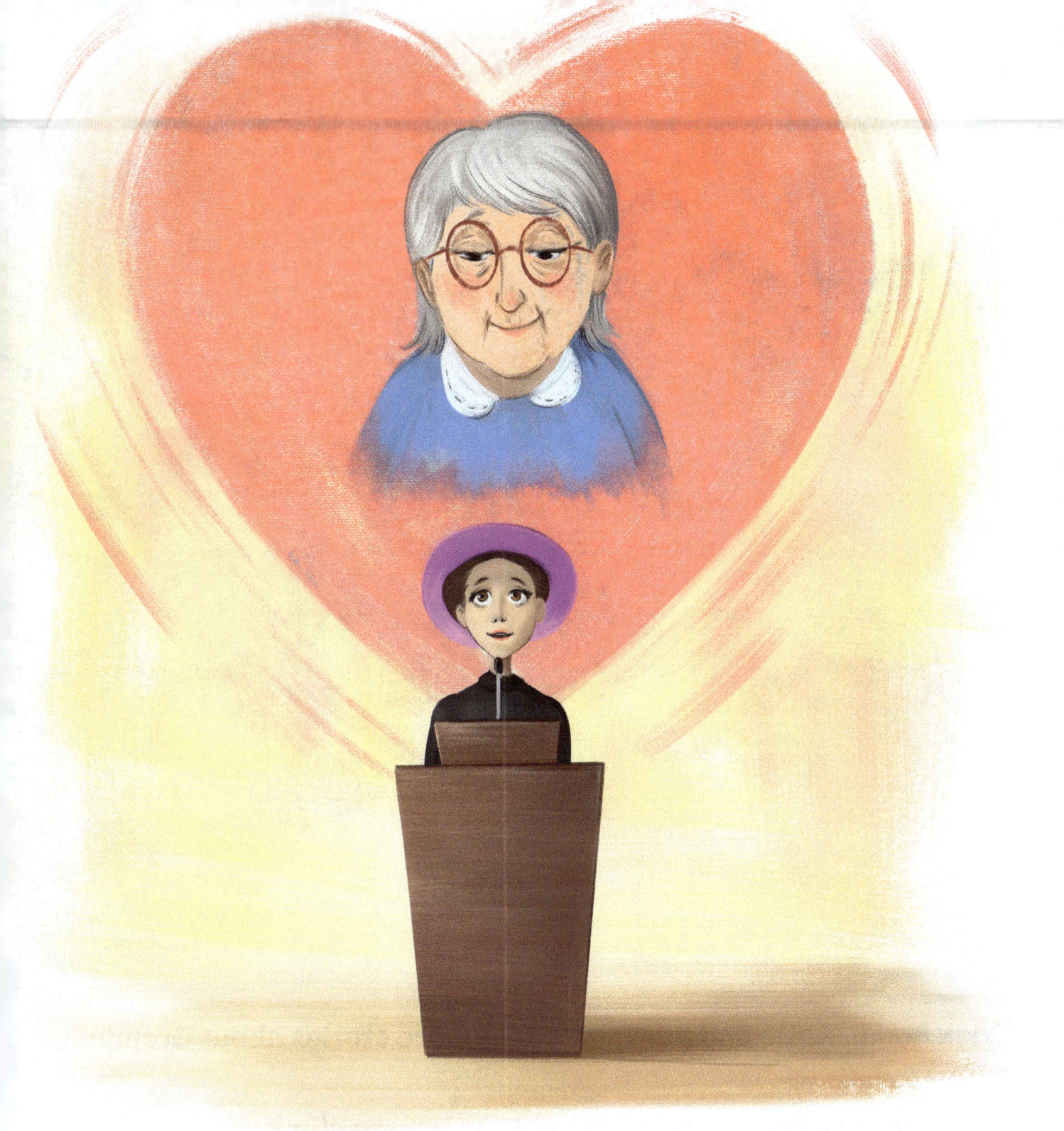

Katie's mummy stood up and told everyone how she remembered her mom. 'She always made big yummy meals for us, and she always helped us with our homework. She worked so hard and always had a smile for us when things were rough.'

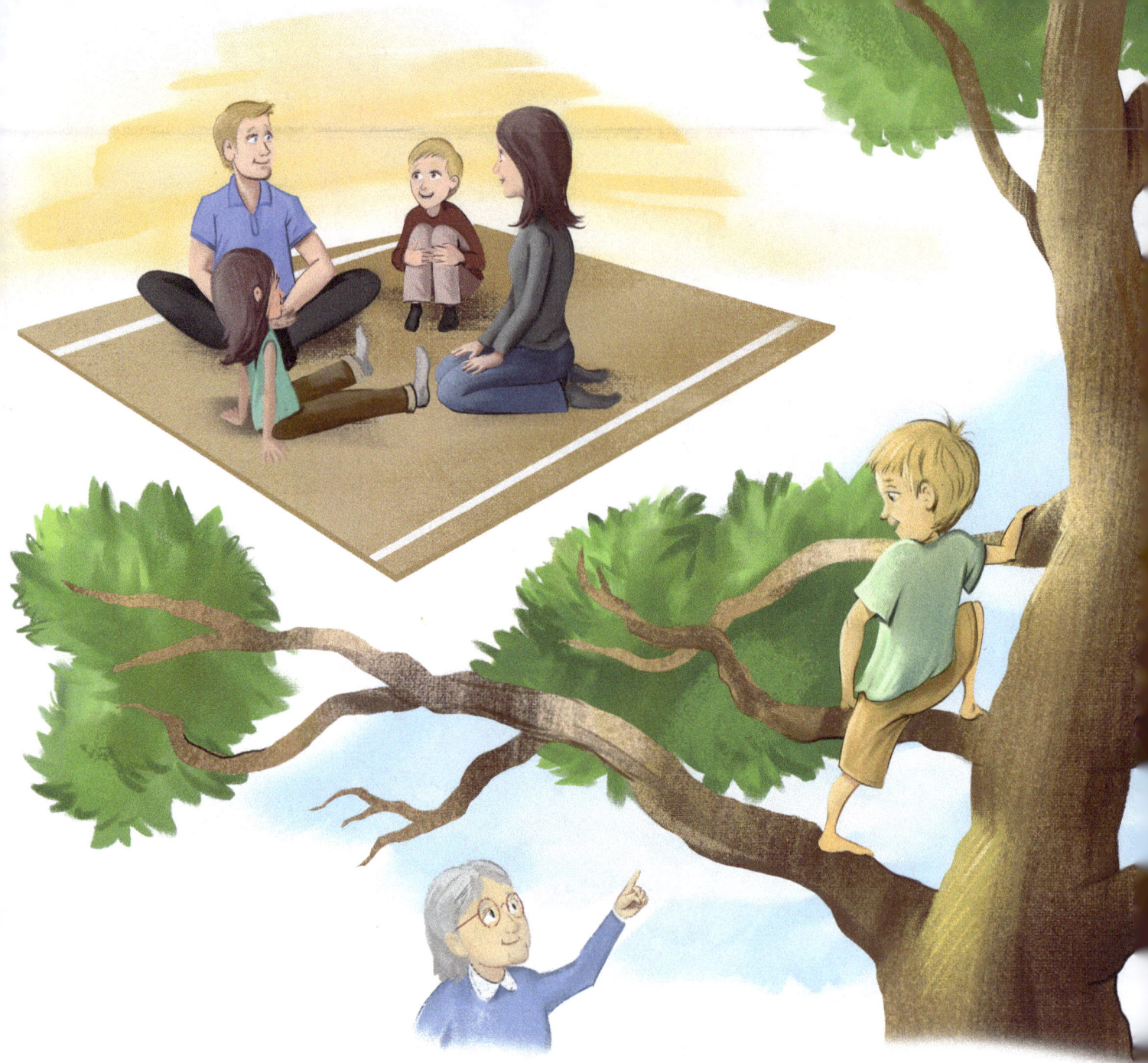

Back home, Katie and her family told more stories about Grandma.

'I remember when Grandma taught me how to climb a tree,' said
Richard. 'She told me to check each branch before I stood on it, or
held on to it, to make sure it won't break!'

Everyone smiled.

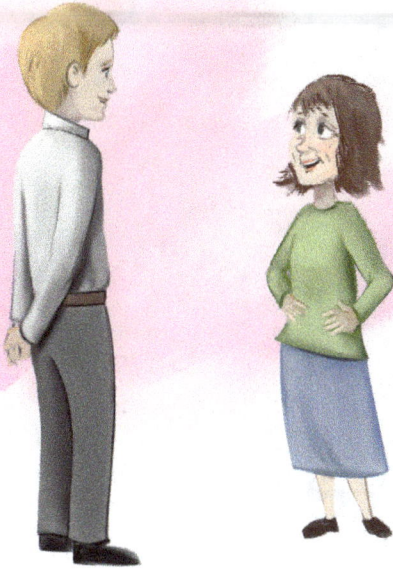

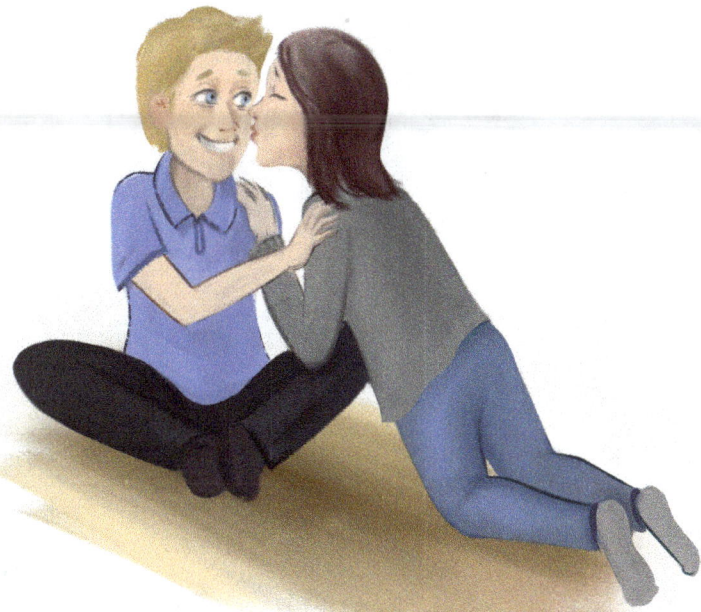

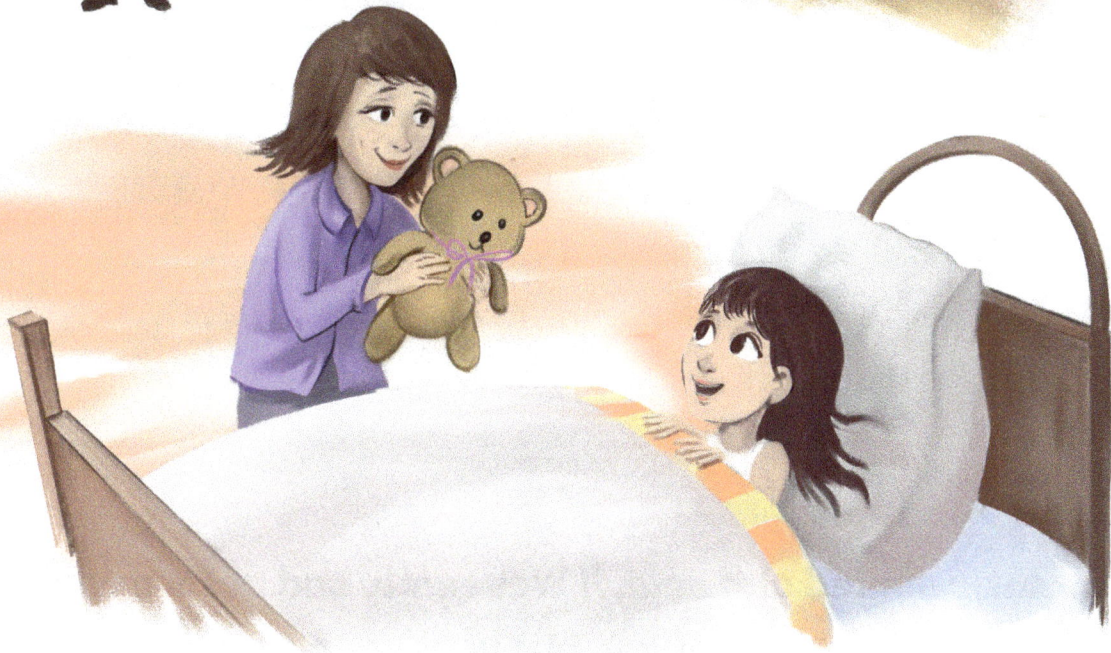

Daddy said, 'I remember when I told Grandma I was going to marry your mom. She told me I'd better be good to Mummy, or I'd be in trouble.'

Everyone laughed, and Mummy kissed Daddy on the cheek.

Mummy said, 'I remember when I was sick when I was little, and Grandma gave me a small stuffed bear. She was always so kind and sweet.'

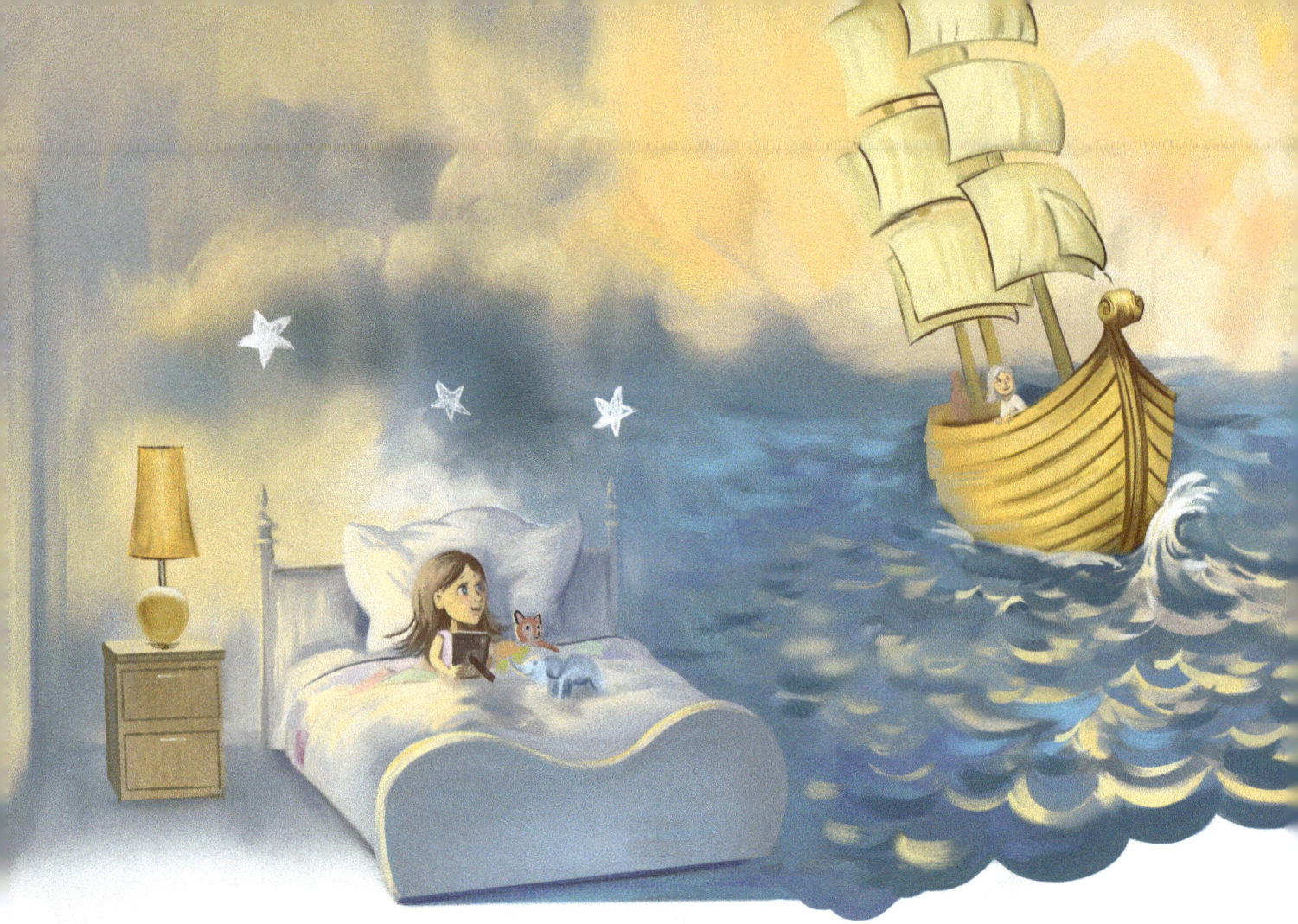

Katie smiled and said, 'I was really sad before when you told me Grandma passed away, but now I don't know. I feel almost happy but sad at the same time. I miss her, but she was so good, and she helped so many people. It makes me want to be just like her.'

And so, that night, before she turned off her bedside lamp, Katie looked at a picture of Grandma. Grandma had a sweet smile with dimples on either side of her face. Katie imagined Grandma on that big ship, setting off to sea, and the sun setting as a warm breeze gently blew.

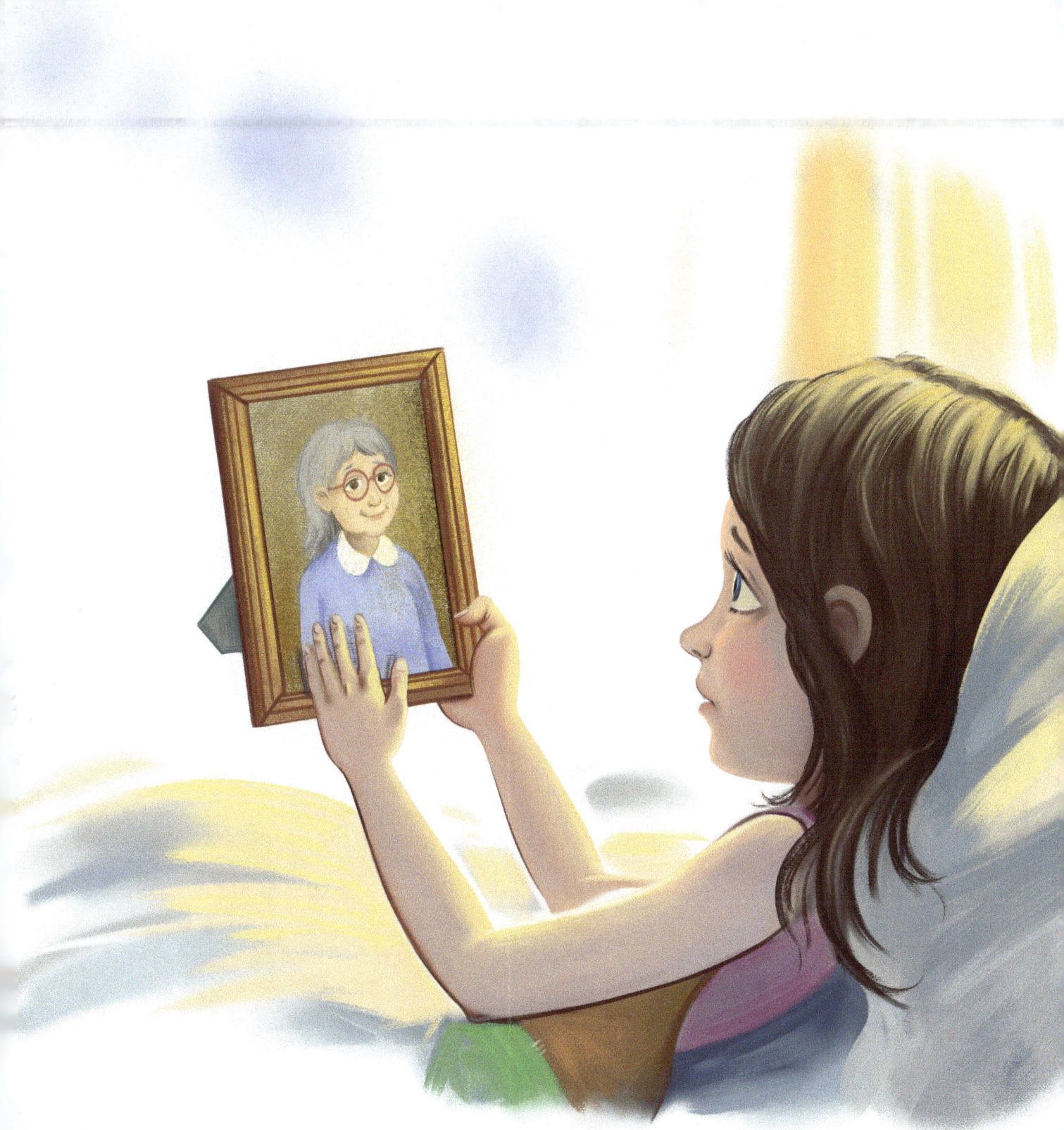

'Goodbye, Grandma,' Katie whispered. 'I'll always love you and remember you. You're always here with me.'

The End!

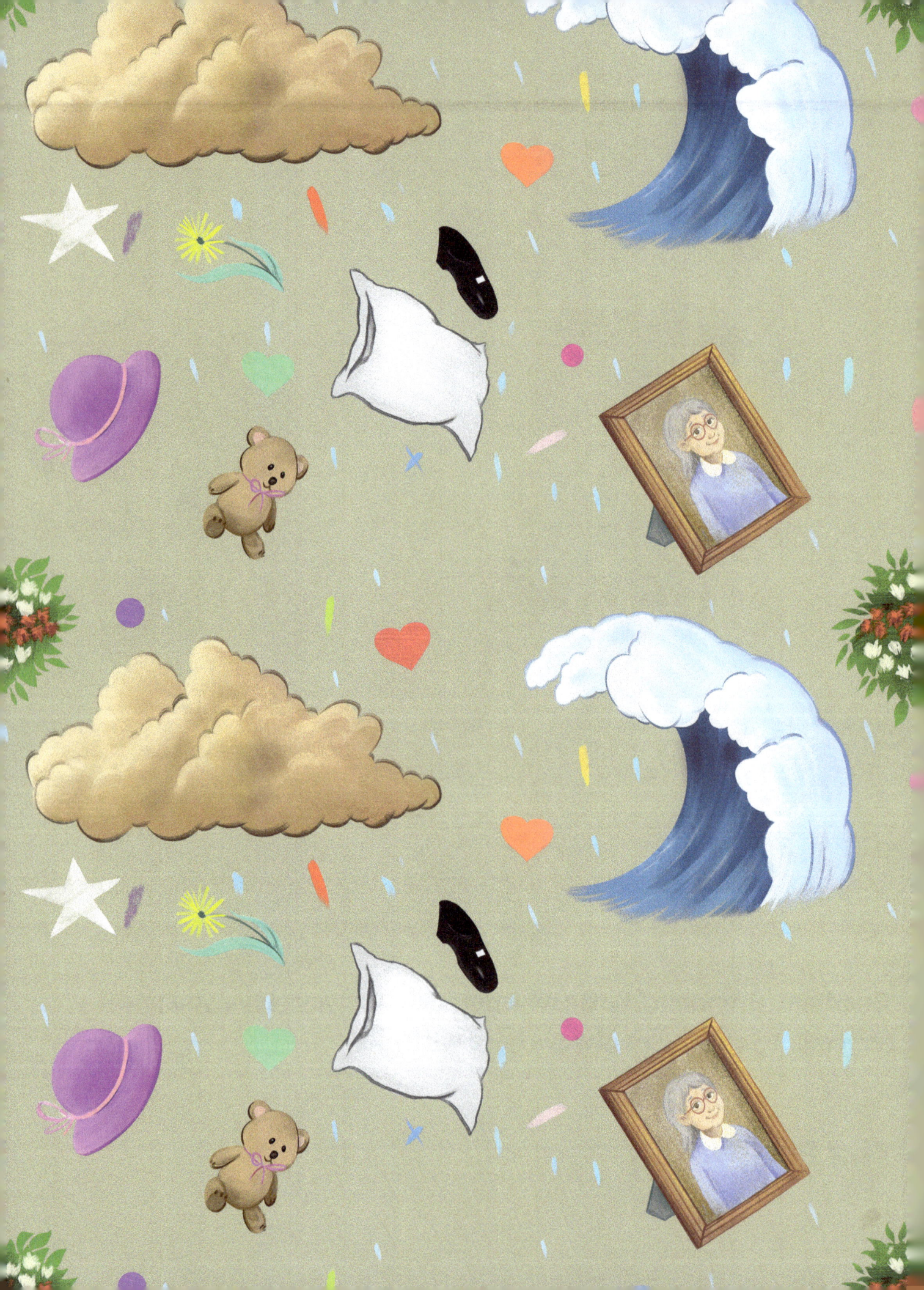

Grandma's Sunset Goodbye is one of several books I have written about the reality of facing cancer, and in this case, it is the gentle passing of a much loved grandparent and how the family comes to terms with their loss.

After I released my first book *The Monster in Mummy*, I became more and more involved with different charities and organisations. Other cancer survivors then started to contact me and telling me their own stories. I realised there is so much we as a society are not aware of especially when it comes to what cancer survivors go through. Their stories are so powerful and yet we hardly heard from patients. Why is that? I am so humble and proud to be able to bring you these stories and help raise awareness that behind every cancer diagnostic is a real person.

Donia Youssef, Author & Producer of *The Monster series*.

www.ingramcontent.com/pod-product-compliance
Lightning Source LLC
Chambersburg PA
CBHW080802300326

41914CB00055B/1026